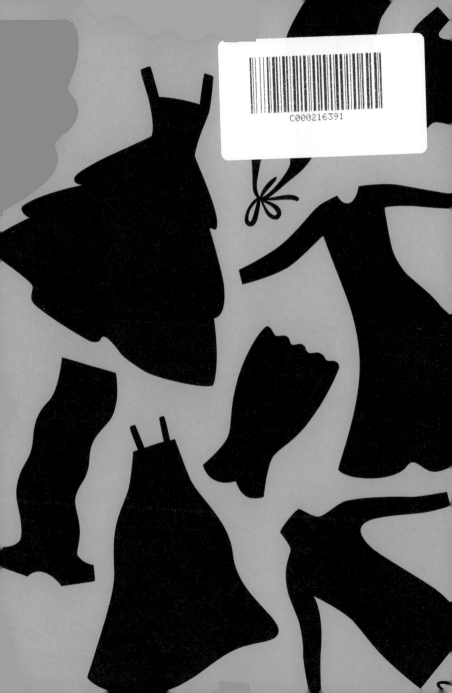

C000216391

THE ART

of the

BLACK

DRESS

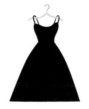

Hardie Grant

BOOKS

CONTENTS

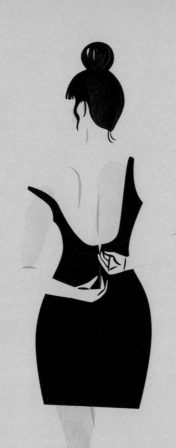

INTRODUCTION

Perhaps the most loved and trusted item in your
wardrobe, the little black dress (or LBD as it's
affectionately known) – made *à la mode* by Coco
Chanel in the 1920s – has a magical suits-all appeal.

As *The Art of the Black Dress* will illustrate, the LBD
is a versatile number, too, and can be worn in a myriad
of individual ways.

From the understated elegance of Audrey Hepburn
to the rock chick cool of Kate Moss via the Paparazzi-
grabbing chutzpah of Liz Hurley, this book charts how
ten iconic women have worked the black dress to suit
their style.

MASTER THE ART OF THE BLACK DRESS!

THE BLACK DRESS IN STYLE

*How the little black dress became
a wardrobe hero*

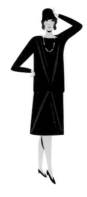

Let's wind back to 1926. The Roaring Twenties were in full roar when *Vogue* featured a simple black *crêpe de chine* dress by designer of the moment, Coco Chanel. Fitted, on-the-knee and with narrow sleeves, the dress was worn simply with a string of pearls. *Vogue* coined it 'Chanel's Ford' and described it as 'a sort of uniform for all women'.

Fellow designers had flirted with the black dress before (nod to Jeanne Lanvin, Elsa Schiaparelli and Jean Patou) but this was the moment the garment was truly delivered to the masses. Boom! The LBD was born. From that day on, the LBD became the byword for effortless glamour.

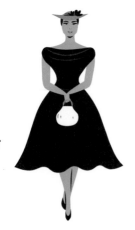

Ever since, the LBD has sashayed its way into every decade. From the timeless elegance of Jacques Fath's 50s hourglass frocks and modish cool of Mary Quant's 60s mini dresses to the body-hugging glamour of Christina Stambolian's 80s cocktail dresses, it's the fall-back going out frock for anyone and everyone.

The ultimate LBD? Arguably Hubert de Givenchy's simple and striking LBDs for Audrey Hepburn in 1961's *Breakfast at Tiffany's*. That iconic image of Hepburn staring into the window of Tiffany's, wearing a sleek black satin gown with a low-cut back, epitomises everything that is good about this perennial wardrobe staple.

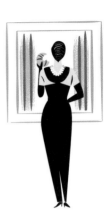

Dress it up or dress it down, from simple everyday office attire to glamorous nights out, the LBD is probably the hardest working item in your wardrobe. As *The Art of the Black Dress* will reveal, it can look equally good with a pair of white Converse as with a pair of dagger-heeled stilettos and diamonds.

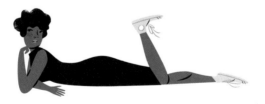

As British designer, Jean Muir, said of the black dress: 'When you have found something that suits you and never lets you down, why not stick to it?' Long live the LBD.

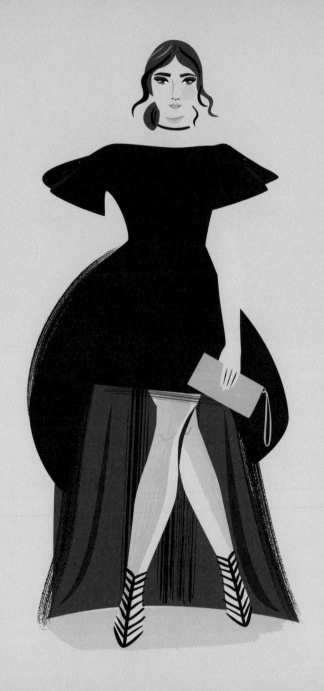

Fluttery Velvet Gown

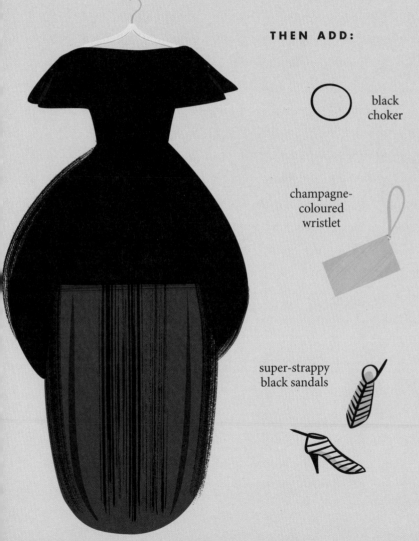

THEN ADD:

black
choker

champagne-
coloured
wristlet

super-strappy
black sandals

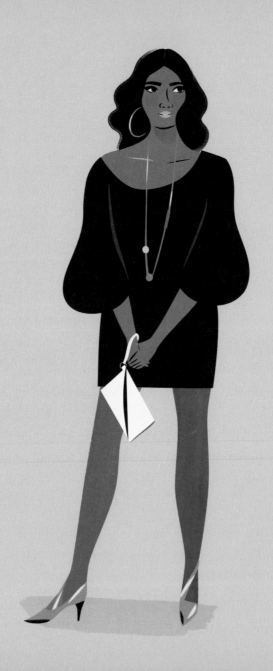

Breezy Linen Minidress

THEN ADD:

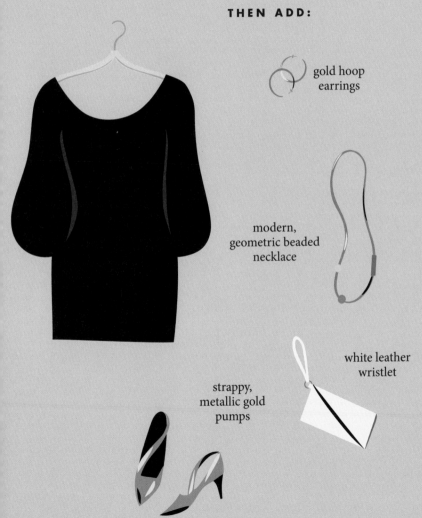

gold hoop
earrings

modern,
geometric beaded
necklace

white leather
wristlet

strappy,
metallic gold
pumps

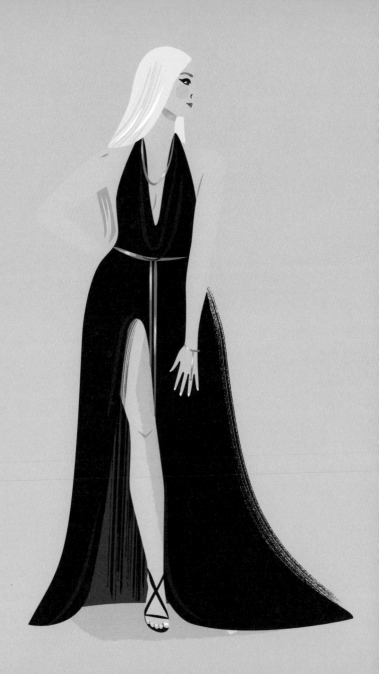

Flowy, Grecian-style Gown with a Dramatic Slit

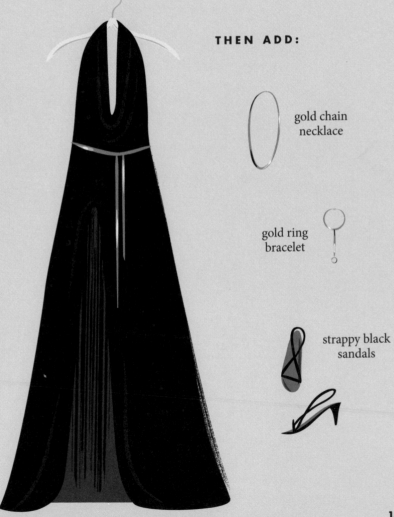

THEN ADD:

gold chain
necklace

gold ring
bracelet

strappy black
sandals

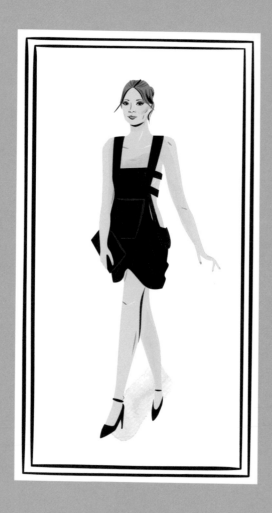

Style Icon

KATE MOSS

Queen of the catwalk. Razor-sharp cheekbones, an impish physique and the sort of innate, effortless style we all wish we had, Kate Moss is the most photographed model on the planet for good reason.

The waifiest of the waifs, was discovered at JFK airport at the tender age of 14, became the face of Calvin Klein at 18 (straddling a buff Mark Wahlberg, no less) and landed first front cover for British *Vogue* at 19.

Born in Croydon in 1974, Kate shot to the height of fashion super stardom at lightening-bolt speed after some no-frills snaps by photographer Corinne Day for *i-D* magazine in 1993. With her nonchalant sense of cool, south London swagger, cheeky laugh and unashamed ability to have fun, Kate become not only the face of the 90s but the embodiment of its party spirit.

From the early days, Kate has also championed the little black dress; in 1998 stepping out with then boyfriend Johnny Depp in a body-skimming vintage cocktail dress adorned with feathers at the Cannes film festival. In 2002, she famously wore a little black apron-style with bandage-like

"In my next life I'm going to be a rock star."

straps by Balenciaga to Mario Testino's private exhibition at the National Portrait Gallery. Sexy yet oozing cool and accessorised by just a white fur coat, a cigarette and a glass of Champagne, it remains one of Kate's coolest – and most Kateish – looks.

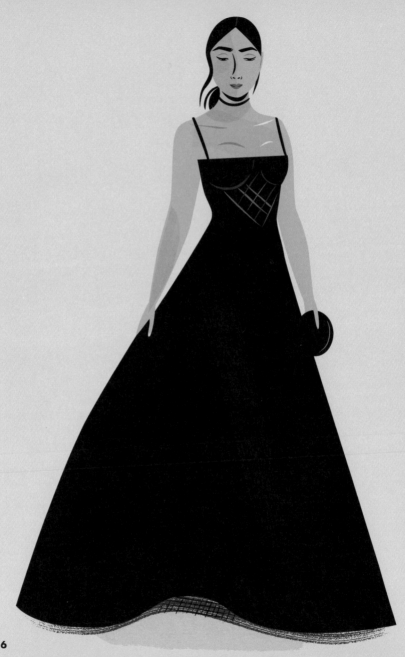

Corseted Leather Gown

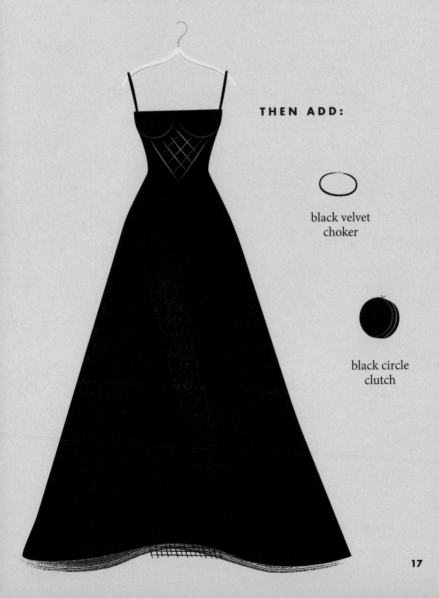

THEN ADD:

black velvet
choker

black circle
clutch

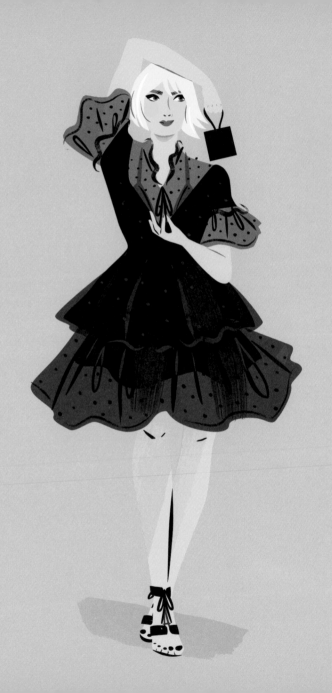

Flouncy, Tiered Chiffon Dress

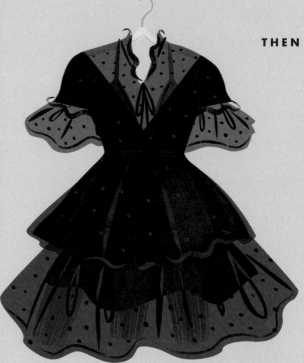

black leather
mini wristlet

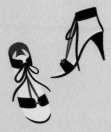

strappy black
lace-up sandals

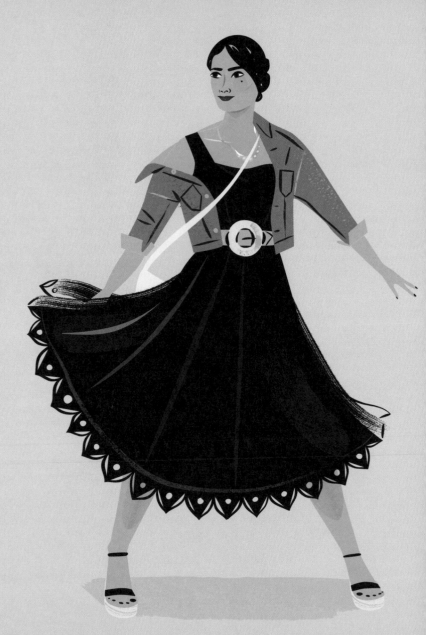

Folksy, Flowing Sundress

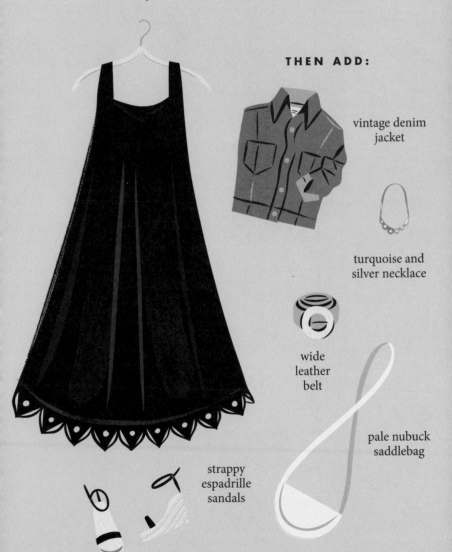

THEN ADD:

vintage denim
jacket

turquoise and
silver necklace

wide
leather
belt

pale nubuck
saddlebag

strappy
espadrille
sandals

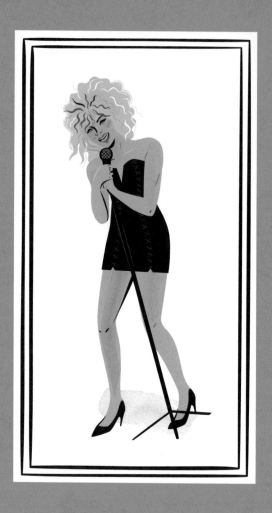

Style Icon

TINA TURNER

Legs of legend, a hairstyle with its own Pinterest board and a soft and gravelly voice like no other, it can only be rock icon Tina Turner. Born Anna Mae Bullock in 1939 and raised by her grandmother in Nutbush, Tennessee, she soon found her musical groove.

Tina brought a new rocky style to St Louis' R&B scene in the 50s. It was during this musically transformative decade that Tina met musician and rock and roll pioneer Ike Turner. Between them, they defined a new style of music that blended classic blues with rock, touring with *The Rolling Stones* in 1969.

After ditching Ike in 1976, Tina went on to forge a solo career while bringing up her two kids (read her autobiography *I, Tina*). In 'Nutbush City Limits' (1973) rock was blended with country music and soul, and people went nuts for it. Fast forward to 1984, Tina established herself as one of the icons of the 1980s when she made it as a solo artist with *Private Dancer*. She went on to sell over 20 million copies worldwide and win four Grammy Awards and a year later starred opposite Mel Gibson in *Mad Max Beyond Thunderdome*.

> *"My greatest beauty secret is being happy with myself."*

During her meteoric rise to music superstardom, Tina rocked a unique stage look: high heels, short hemlines, huge punky wigs and a penchant for short leather black dresses, epitomised by a 1996 D&G corseted leather mini dress she wore to sing James Bond classic *GoldenEye*.

Anything but demure, Tina amped-up the appeal of the little black dress, proving it can be the ultimate symbol for rock and roll attitude. Breaking every rule, as usual Tina.

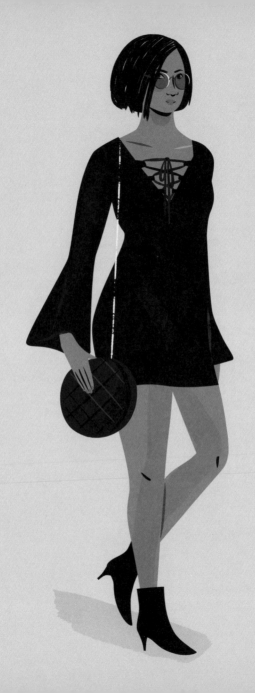

Lace-up Knit Minidress

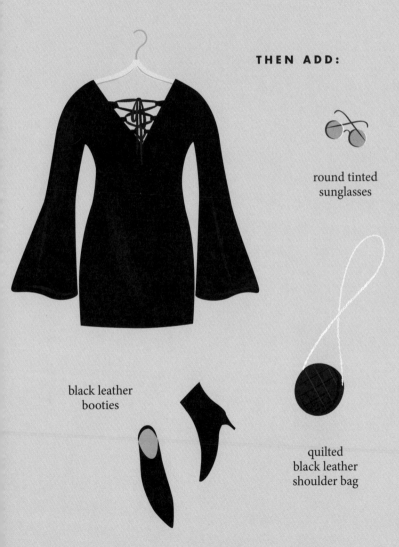

round tinted
sunglasses

black leather
booties

quilted
black leather
shoulder bag

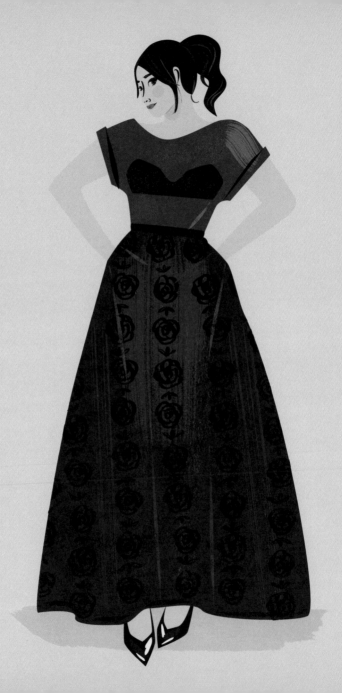

START WITH A

Layered, Flocked Organza Gown

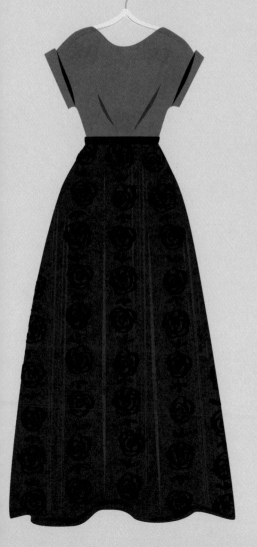

THEN ADD:

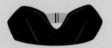

black strapless bra

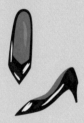

black patent
leather pumps

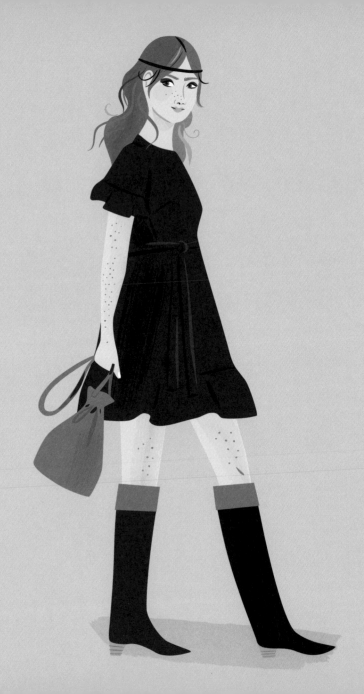

Ruffled, Sashed Wool Crêpe Dress

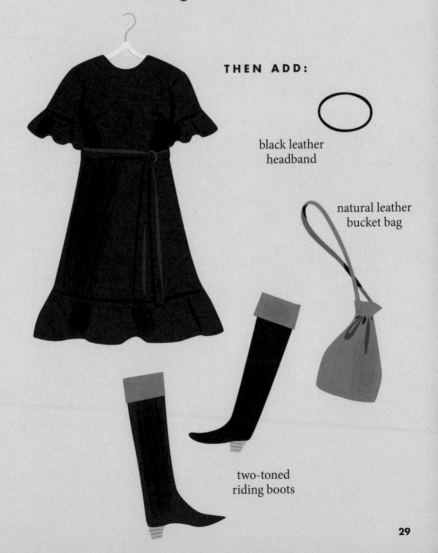

THEN ADD:

black leather
headband

natural leather
bucket bag

two-toned
riding boots

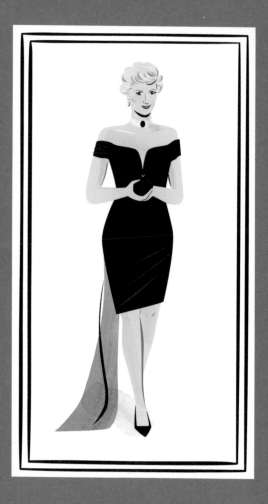

Style Icon

PRINCESS DIANA

With her large khol-rimmed eyes, blonde hair flicks and boxy shoulder pads, Lady Diana Spencer (1961–1997) epitomised British 80s glamour.

The young Diana Frances Spencer was a Sloane Ranger icon, known for her simple, preppy style – think ballerina flats, polka dots and Peter Pan collars – all worn with fluttering lashes and a coy smile.

When Lady Di married Prince Charles at St Paul's Cathedral in 1981 wearing an ivory silk taffeta gown with a 25 feet (7.6 metres) train by David and Elizabeth Emanuel, she looked every inch the fairytale princess. However, beneath the smiles was a loveless marriage which would end up producing one of the killer LBD moments in history.

As Princess Di's marriage faded, her style sharpened. Her signature going-out look became the off-the-shoulder black cocktail dress worn with a choker, pearl earrings and stilettos. The ultimate? The post-divorce 'revenge' dress by Christina Stambolian she wore to the Serpentine gallery party in 1994.

> *"Only do what your heart tells you."*

Princess Di became a devoted mother to princes William and Harry, patron of the arts and charities, passionate about humanitarian causes and earned her the name 'the people's princess'. Her style evolved with the help of a clutch of loyal designers including Catherine Walker, Bruce Oldfield and Victor Edelstein.

Diana's death at the age of just 36 in 1997 remains one of the most shocking – and tragic – moments of the 20th century. Her light lives on.

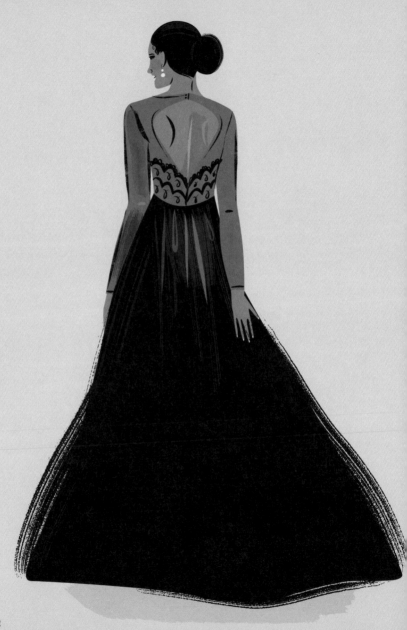

Open-backed Dramatic Gown

THEN ADD:

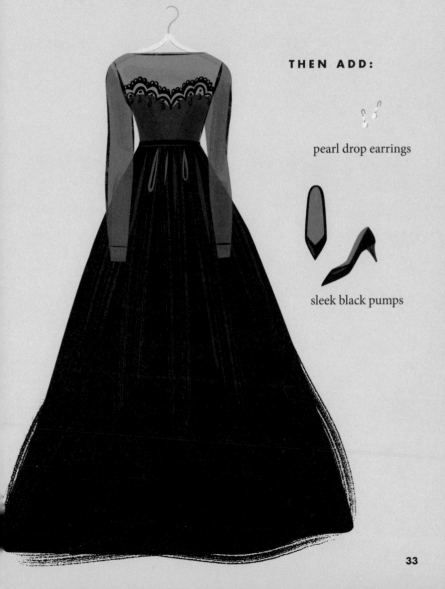

pearl drop earrings

sleek black pumps

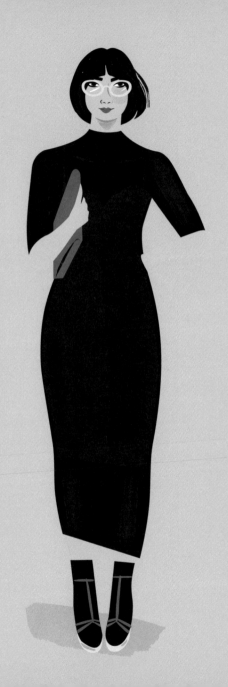

Clingy, Sheer, Layered Dress

THEN ADD:

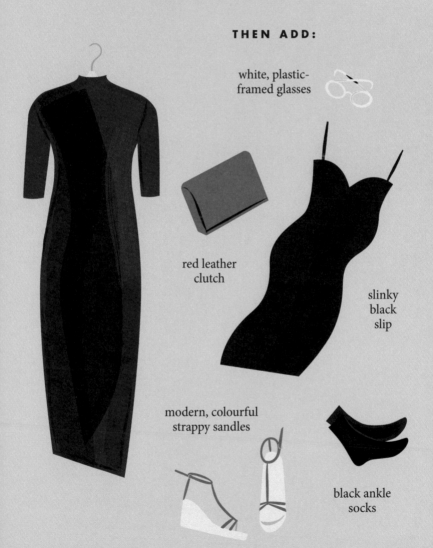

white, plastic-
framed glasses

red leather
clutch

slinky
black
slip

modern, colourful
strappy sandles

black ankle
socks

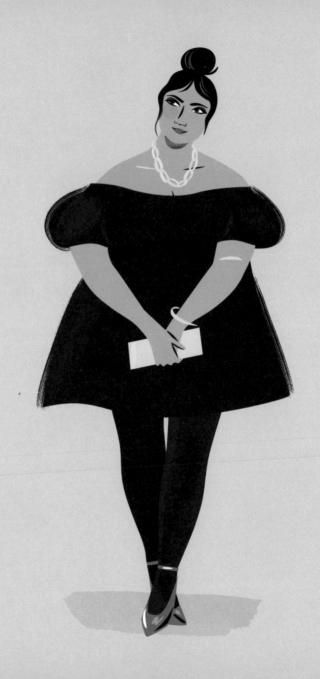

Off-the-shoulder Velvet Minidress

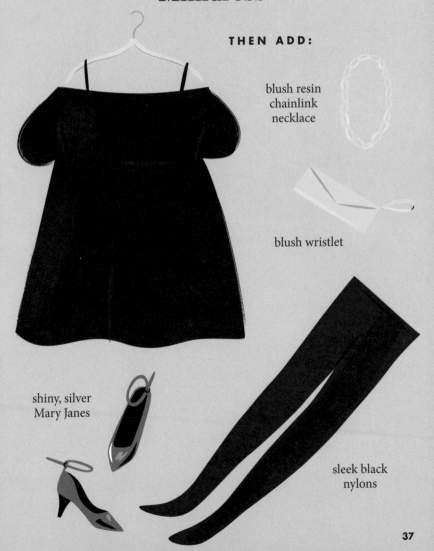

blush resin chainlink necklace

blush wristlet

shiny, silver Mary Janes

sleek black nylons

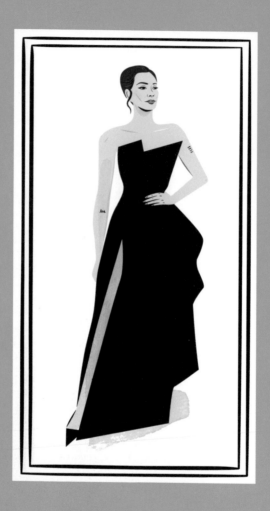

Style Icon

ANGELINA JOLIE

From gothy Hollywood kid to mother-of-six and UN Goodwill ambassador, few actresses have transformed their image in such dramatic style as Angelina Jolie.

Born in LA in 1975, the daughter of actor Jon Voight and actress and humanitarian Marcheline Bertand, the Hollywood thoroughbred has been in the spotlight from day one.

With her chiselled cheekbones, bee-stung pout and perfectly-proportioned figure, Jolie, has topped every 'sexiest women' and 'most beautiful women' list out there. Her break-through film was *Girl Interrupted* in which she masterfully played a mentally-ill patient and off-screen did everything to perpetuate an offbeat, kooky image.

Jolie became a poster girl for post-modern female power when she starred as kick-ass adventurer in *Lara Croft: Tomb Raider* in 2001, in which she performed all her own stunts.

From the beginning, Jolie has known the power of black, wearing it for most of her red carpet appearances and perhaps most famously when she was snapped in the iconic Versace dress with a leg-revealing slit for the Oscars in 2012.

"Make bold choices and make mistakes. It's all these things that add up to the person you become."

Over the years, Jolie has turned heads in a succession of LBDs by designers including Elie Saab, Armani and Tom Ford and a body hugging black leather dress for the premiere of *Mr and Mrs Smith*, in which she starred alongside Brad Pitt. And we all know what happened next...

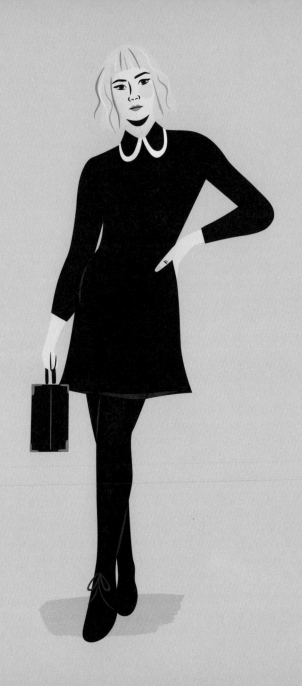

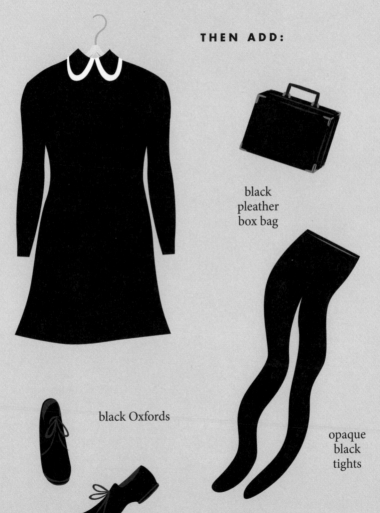

Minidress with
a Peterpan Collar

THEN ADD:

black
pleather
box bag

black Oxfords

opaque
black
tights

41

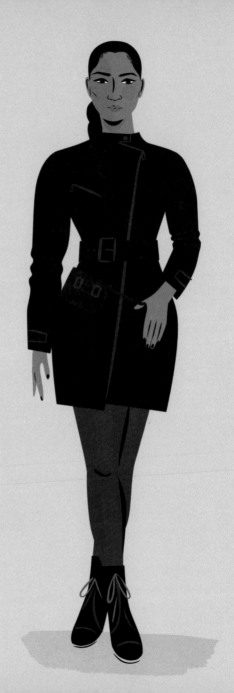

Leather Jacket Dress

THEN ADD:

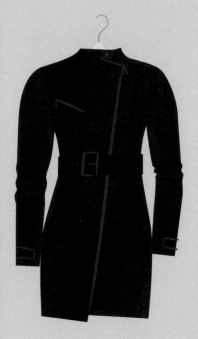

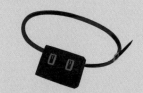

black leather
bum bag

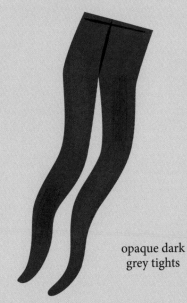

opaque dark
grey tights

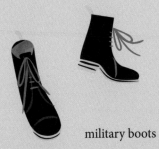

military boots

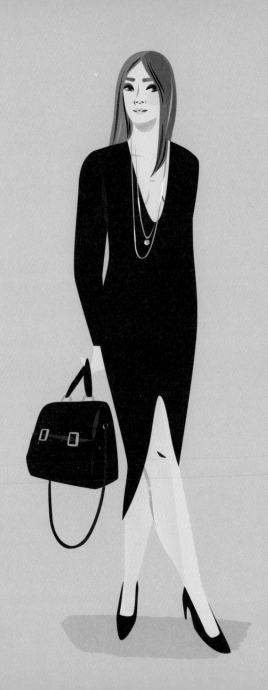

Low-cut, Slitted
Sheath Dress

THEN ADD:

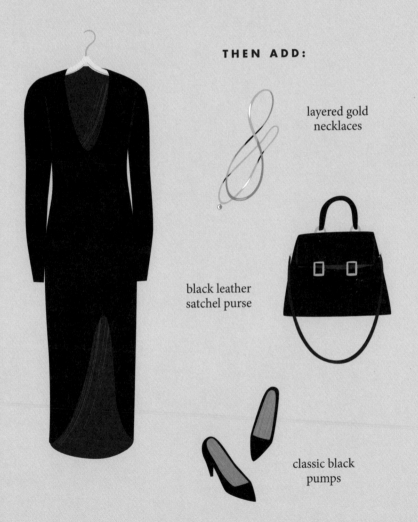

layered gold
necklaces

black leather
satchel purse

classic black
pumps

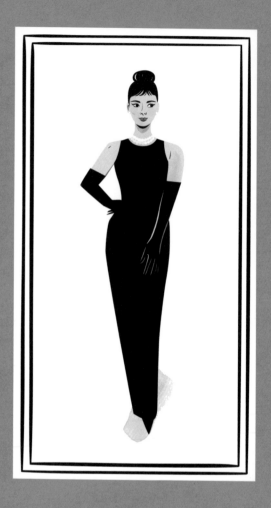

Style Icon

AUDREY HEPBURN

Speaker of five languages, a trained ballerina and one of only a handful of stars to get an EGOT (an Emmy, Grammy, Oscar and Tony award), Audrey Hepburn (1929–1993) will always be one of the world's greatest style icons.

And no wonder, the actress/humanitarian exuded grace and poise like no other. Her simple, tailored, gamine look soon turned heads when she made her London stage debut in 1948 – just three years later she starred in Broadway and was making iconic films with big name directors like Billy Wilder and Stanley Donen.

Born in Belgium in 1929, Hepburn grew up in the UK and moved to the Netherlands during World War 2 before training as a ballerina in Amsterdam. It was when filming *Sabrina*, her second film for Paramount, she requested that designer of the moment Hubert de Givenchy create the costumes. Together they forged a new aesthetic, a world away from the curvy housewife looks of the 1950s. It was sharp, streamlined and extremely chic. And black dresses – a symbol of the daring, avant-garde woman – were intrinsic to this.

"If clothes maketh the man, then costumes certainly make actors and actresses."

Perhaps one of Hollywood's most iconic images ever is the sleek, floor-length black dress Givenchy designed for her character Holly Golightly in *Breakfast at Tiffany's*. Accompanied by long satin gloves, a cigarette holder, sunglasses and diamonds and pearls, that look was the epitome of modern glamour.

Audrey proved, get the silhouette right and the rest follows. 'Givenchy's creations always gave me a sense of security and confidence, and my work went more easily in the knowledge that I looked absolutely right,' she said.

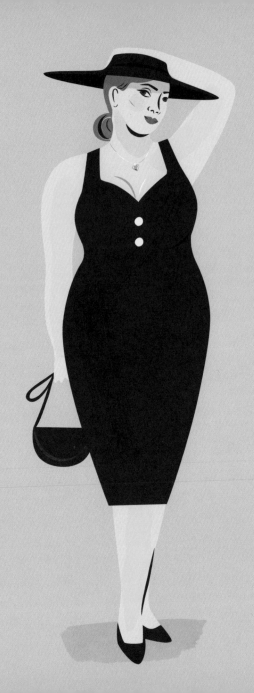

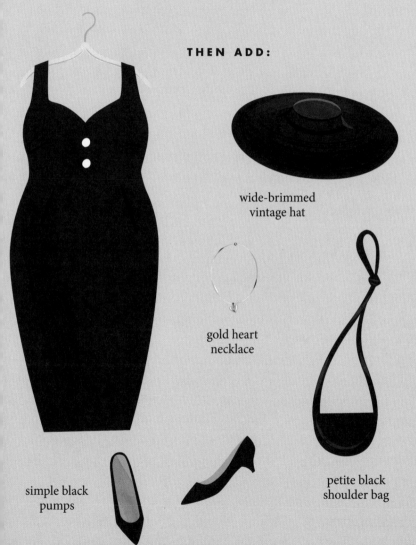

Pencil Dress

THEN ADD:

wide-brimmed
vintage hat

gold heart
necklace

simple black
pumps

petite black
shoulder bag

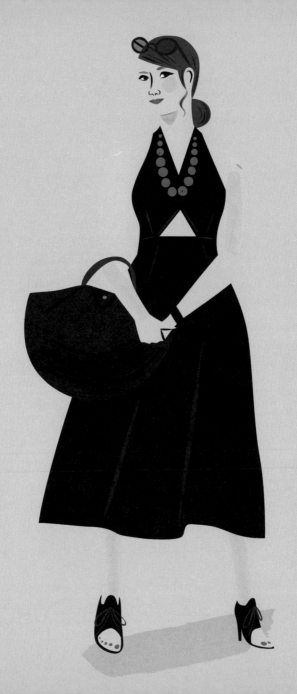

Cotton Halter Sundress

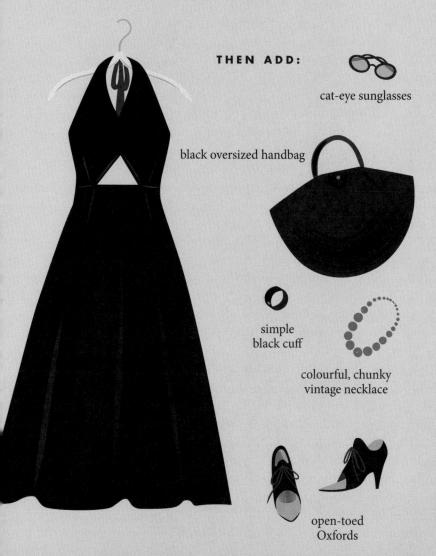

THEN ADD:

cat-eye sunglasses

black oversized handbag

simple
black cuff

colourful, chunky
vintage necklace

open-toed
Oxfords

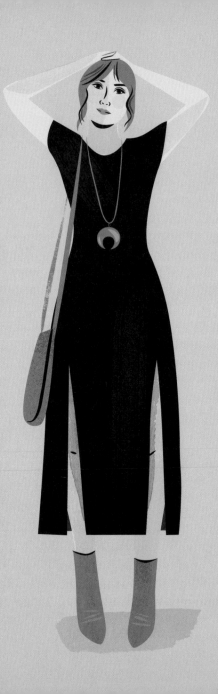

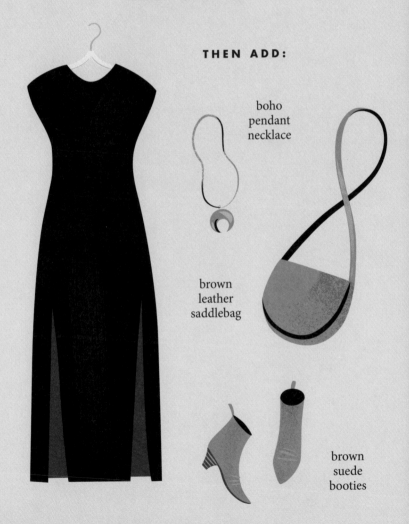

START WITH A

Boho Cotton Slitted Knit Dress

THEN ADD:

boho
pendant
necklace

brown
leather
saddlebag

brown
suede
booties

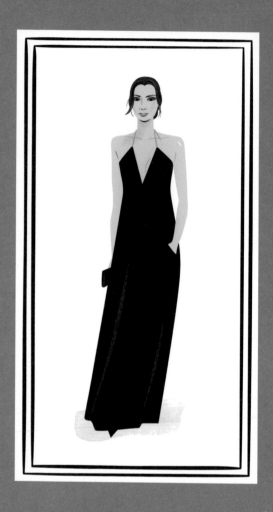

Style Icon
—
VICTORIA BECKHAM

Warm, witty and owner of the sharpest sense of style we know, the former Spice Girl and mother-of-four is queen of the pulled-together look.

There are very few who soar to the top of the fashion food chain with such force, but Victoria Beckham's rise from Posh Spice to seriously-posh designer has been meteoric.

Born Victoria Caroline Adams in 1974 in Harlow, Essex, VB was brought up in leafy Goffs Oak, Hertfordshire, where she idolised Sandy from *Grease* from her Laura Ashley-papered bedroom and was driven to school in her dad's Rolls Royce.

The petite designer, famed for her good humour and strong work ethic, made the transition from Spice Girl to a designer to be reckoned with a quiet determination. Her debut catwalk show for Spring/Summer 2009 was a collection of immaculate, elegant and wearable dresses (and at least a dozen dream LBDs) that wowed the world's fashion editors.

"I'm not a supermodel. I make the most of what I've got."

Even before she entered the world of design, VB's natural sass and clear devotion to fashion had the world's leading designers including Marc Jacobs, Donatella Versace and Roland Mouret courting the pop princess. In 2007 Donatella flew VB to Milan to watch the Versace show where she sat in the front row in an off-the-shoulder black leather dress that defined her super-feminine and structured style.

Victoria has been an avid fan of the LBD before and since, graduating from the miniscule teeny weeny Lycra-body-hugger variety to lean and chic red-carpet show stoppers like the pleated black halter neck she wore for the British Fashion Awards in 2011.

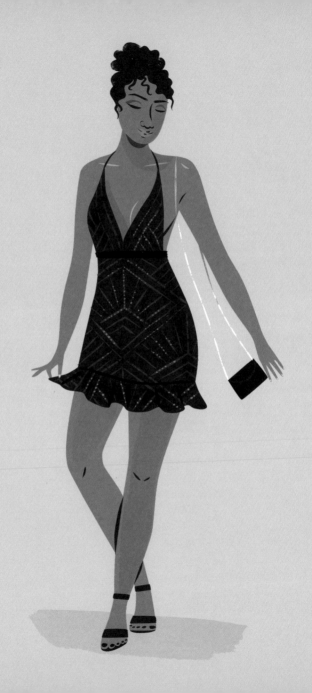

Sexy, Sparkly Cocktail Dress

THEN ADD:

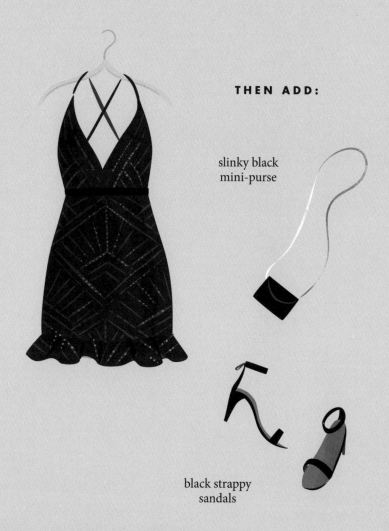

slinky black
mini-purse

black strappy
sandals

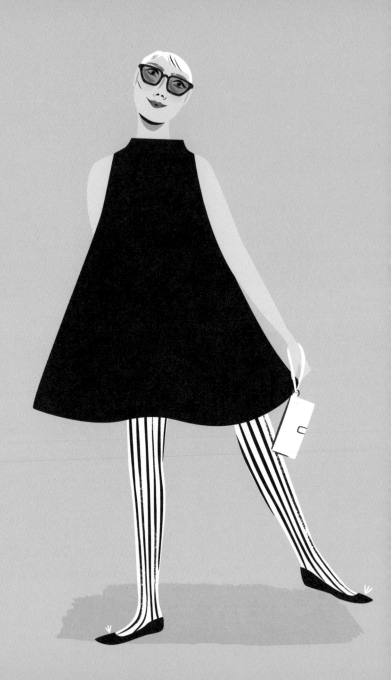

Mod, A-line Minidress

THEN ADD:

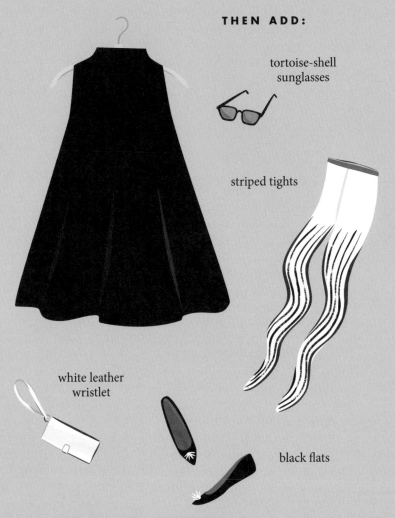

tortoise-shell
sunglasses

striped tights

white leather
wristlet

black flats

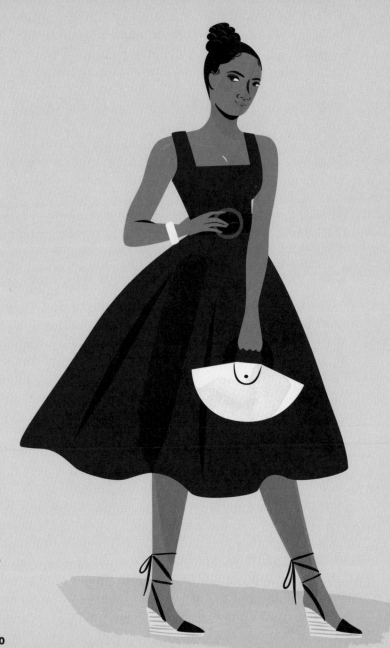

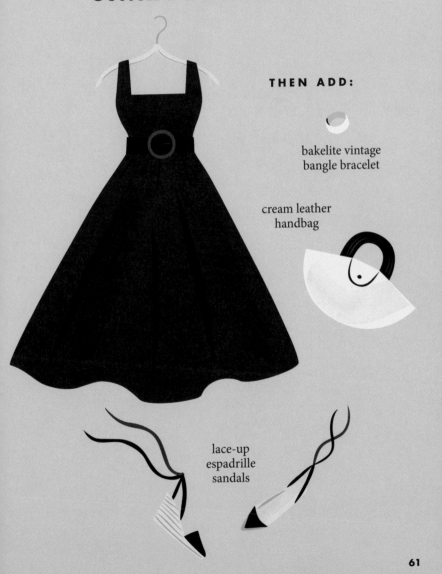

Cotton Full-circle Dress

THEN ADD:

bakelite vintage
bangle bracelet

cream leather
handbag

lace-up
espadrille
sandals

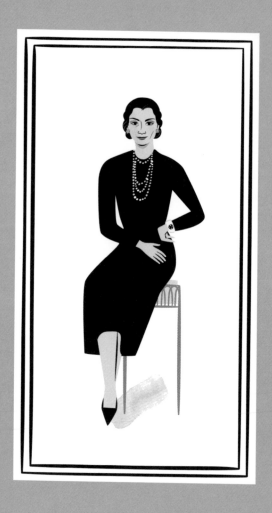

Style Icon

COCO CHANEL

Dresser of stars and the designer that helped emancipate women, Gabrielle Chanel (1883–1971), revolutionised the way modern women dressed in the 20th century. There are many iconic fashion moments we can say a big *merci beaucoup* to Chanel for: the simple chemise, wide-legged trousers, the quilted bag and, of course, the little black dress.

Born in Saumur, near the River Loire, France, the daughter of a laundry woman and merchant, Gabrielle Bonheur Chanel, spent her teens in a convent orphanage where she learned to sew. She worked as a seamstress and cabaret singer (where she earned the nickname 'Coco') before launching her fashion empire.

A natural beauty with a keen eye for design, Chanel had a steely determination and a few male admirers including textile heir Etienne Balsan, who helped fund her first shop; a hat shop in Paris in 1910. (She later opened her first fashion boutique on Rue Cambon, where it remains today.)

In 1914 Chanel created a simple chemise dress that put a middle finger up to the restricting corsets women had been wearing until then. While purveying a more natural, yet still exquisitely chic and put-together silhouette, Chanel invented the Little Black Dress.

"A girl should be two things: classy and fabulous."

Her version? A simple, boxy shift with a higher hemline than had ever been worn. It was a dress that would suit almost anyone and no-one modelled it better than Coco herself. Formidable. Iconoclastic. Feminist. Chanel's LBD set the tone for the style of the next century.

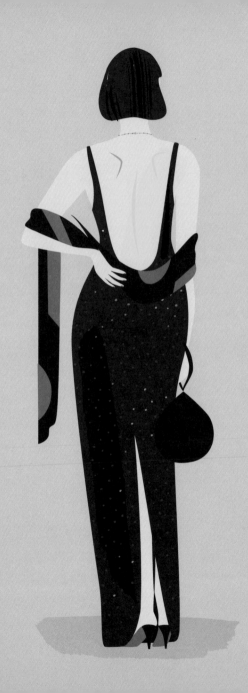

Backless, Sparkly, Slinky Gown

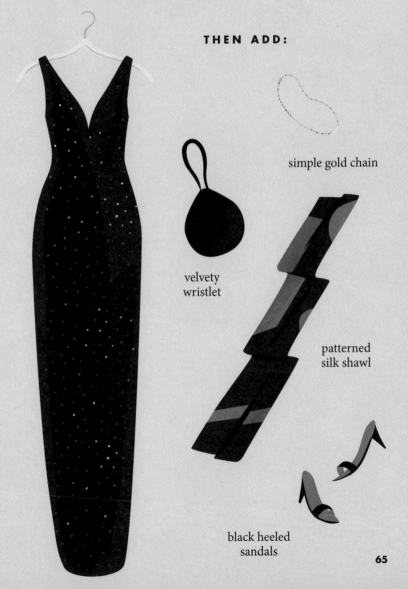

simple gold chain

velvety
wristlet

patterned
silk shawl

black heeled
sandals

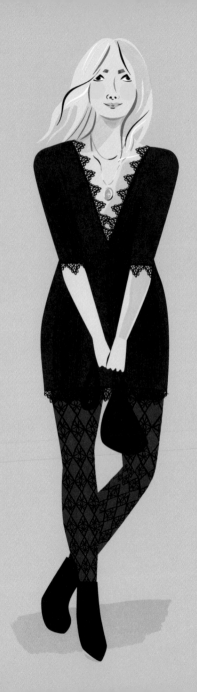

Lace-trimmed Minidress

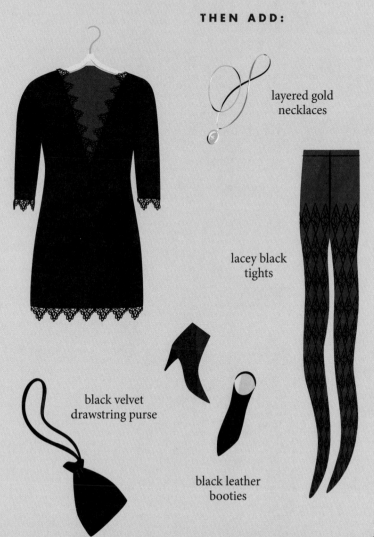

layered gold
necklaces

lacey black
tights

black velvet
drawstring purse

black leather
booties

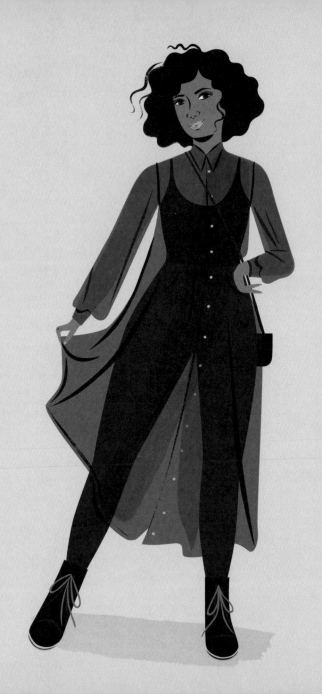

Full-length, Sheer Shirtdress

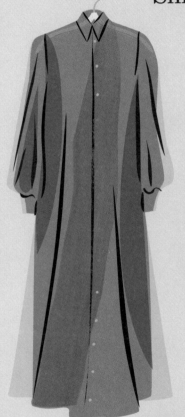

THEN ADD:

slinky black
bodysuit

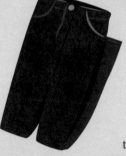

black skinny
jeans

tiny black
cross-body purse

combat boots

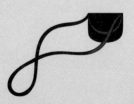

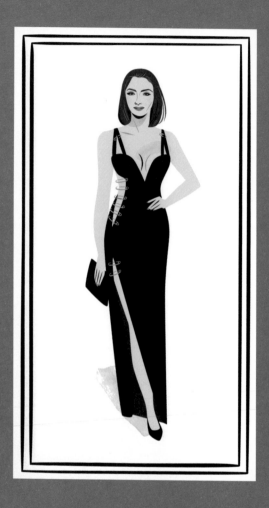

Style Icon

ELIZABETH HURLEY

If we had to choose the most attention-grabbing LBD of all time, there would be no contest: it would be the safety-pinned Versace dress that Elizabeth Hurley wore in 1994 to the premiere of *Four Weddings and a Funeral*, with then boyfriend, Hugh Grant.

With her race-horse toned body saucily, yet somehow also classily, flashed enough cleavage, leg and torso (bound by giant golden safety pins) to make all the newspaper front pages, and ensure her lifelong fame from then on. It's no surprise the dress is still referenced and talked about to this day, has its very own *Wikipedia* page and boasts an appearance on an episode of *The Simpsons*.

Born in 1965 in Basingstoke, Hampshire, Hurley graduated from teenage punk to an aspiring actress starring in films *Austin Powers* and TV series *Gossip Girl*. With her glossy locks, haughty poise, incredible legs and regular society magazine appearances, Hurley epitomised the well-bred Brit model look.

In 1995 Hurley became the face of Estée Lauder and remains the face of its breast cancer campaign. These days, as well as designing and modelling for her eponymous swimwear collection, which she launched in 2005, Hurley can be found hanging out at her Herefordshire country pile with her beloved lookalike son Damian.

"I always wear make-up as I've never seen the point of looking less than your best."

Liz teaches us to never underestimate the power of that well-planned little black dress to dazzle.

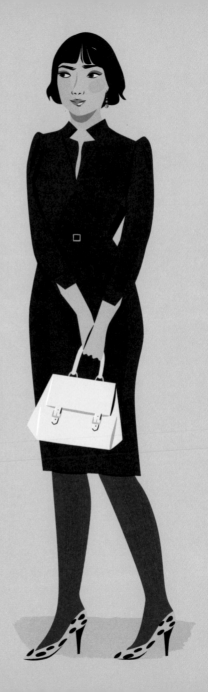

START WITH A

Collared Sheath Dress

THEN ADD:

gold drop earrings

blush leather satchel

grey tights

leopard-print pumps

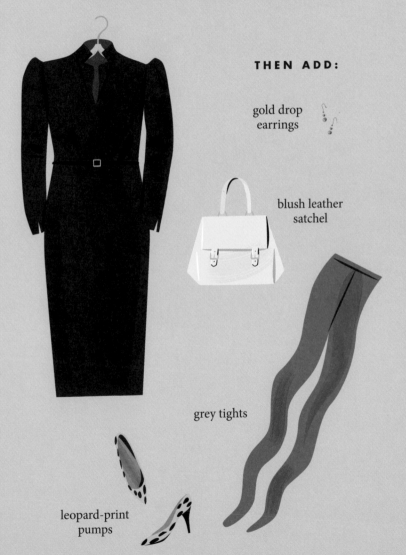

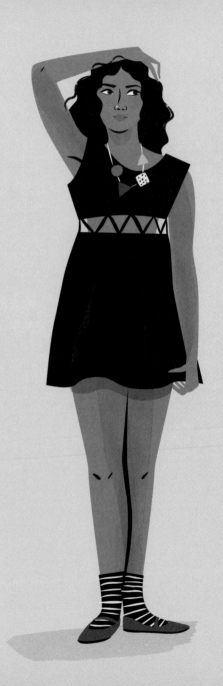

START WITH A

Boho, Suede Minidress

THEN ADD:

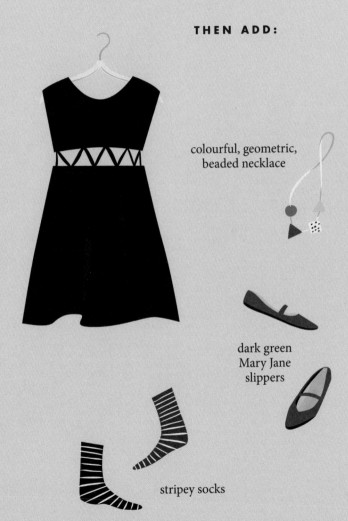

colourful, geometric,
beaded necklace

dark green
Mary Jane
slippers

stripey socks

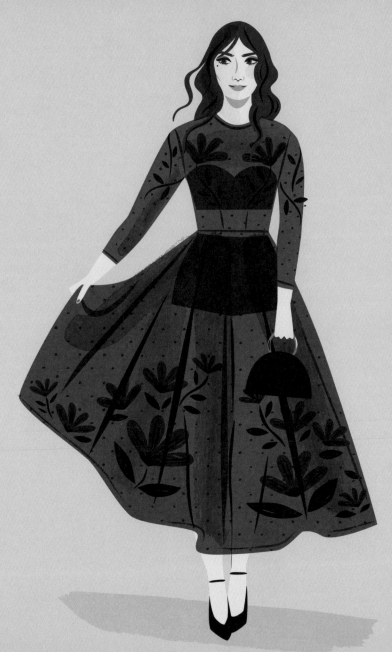

Sheer, Embroidered Gown

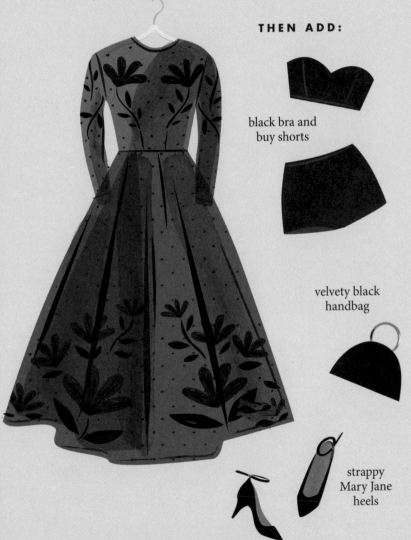

black bra and
buy shorts

velvety black
handbag

strappy
Mary Jane
heels

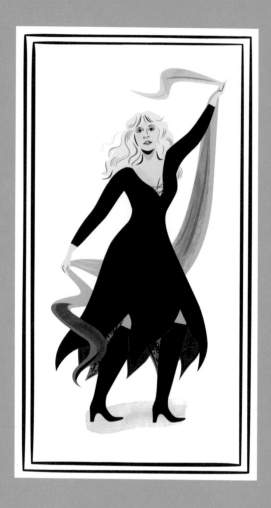

Style Icon
—

STEVIE NICKS

Bell sleeves, billowing dresses, top hats and waistcoats, welcome to the beguiling, witchy-cool world of Stevie Nicks. The original bohemian icon, Nicks has been rocking her very own aesthetic on stage since she joined Fleetwood Mac with then boyfriend Lindsey Buckingham in 1975.

Born in 1948, in Phoenix, Arizona, Stephanie Lynn Nicks, was taught to sing age four by her grandfather, Aaron Jess Nicks, a country singer. On being given a Goya guitar for her 16th birthday, she started writing songs and the rest is rock and roll history.

Stevie has spent her stage career layering lace and leather in a gypsy-cool way which LA-based stylist Margi Kent help her evolve. She recently revealed she has a temperature-controlled vault for her vast collection of shawls. Along with shawls, for Nicks, the black dress has been a vehicle for self-expression, a free, floaty, wispy canvas that encapsulates her free spirit style and has inspired designers including Rodarte, Anna Sui and Ralph Lauren.

"I'll never be in style, but I'll always be different."

When Nicks launched her solo career with the song 'Bella Donna' in 1981, she wore a black dress with lace sleeves for the vinyl inset, photographed alongside fellow-vocalists Sharon Celani and Lori Perry in a smouldering pose.

Nicks, a lifelong fan of black said: 'Halloween is my favourite day, but I never have to wonder: what am I gonna be for Halloween this year? A witch, of course. Wearing my Stevie Nicks clothes.' Us too, Stevie, us too.

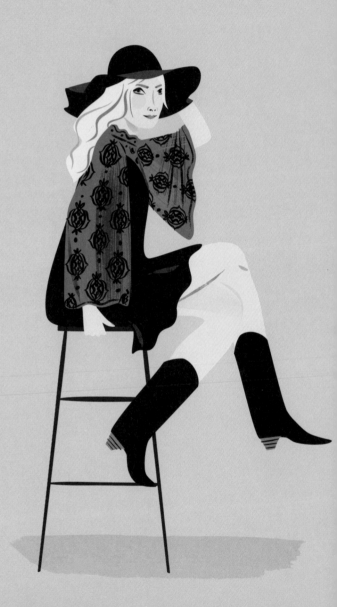

Bell-sleeved Baby Doll Dress

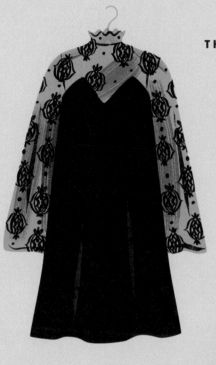

THEN ADD:

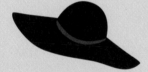

floppy, black
brimmed hat

black cowboy boots

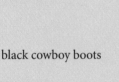

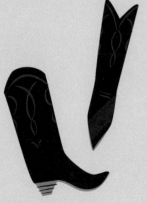

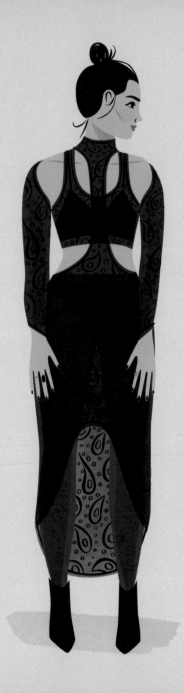

Futuristic Nylon, Cut-out Dress

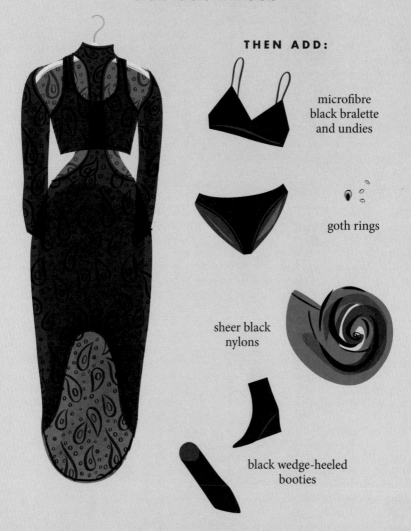

THEN ADD:

microfibre
black bralette
and undies

goth rings

sheer black
nylons

black wedge-heeled
booties

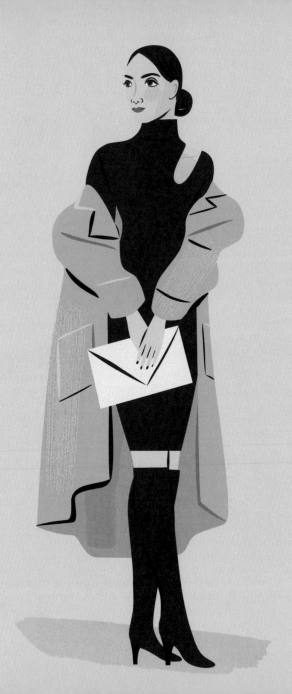

START WITH A

Turtleneck Cut-out Dress

THEN ADD:

camel-coloured
wool trench

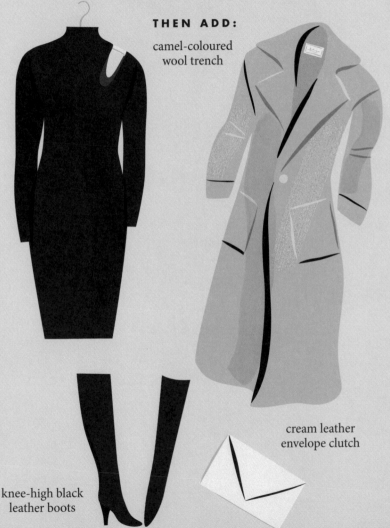

cream leather
envelope clutch

knee-high black
leather boots

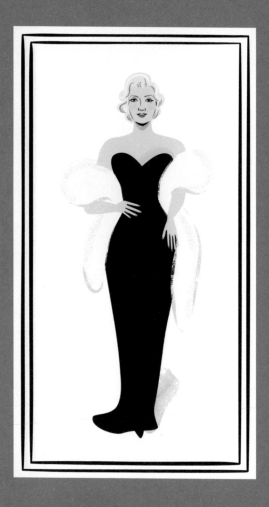

Style Icon

MARILYN MONROE

The baby blonde locks, the china-doll complexion, the well-placed beauty spot, those plump red lips and that hourglass figure; was there ever a sexier human on earth? But Marilyn's sexbomb persona was tinged with sadness.

Born Norma Jeane Mortenson in Los Angeles in 1926, her mother Gladys Pearl Baker, a film-cutter in LA, had mental illness and spent time in hospital. Marilyn never knew her father and she spent her childhood in and out of foster homes. At 16 she married aircraft plane worker, James Dougherty, to escape her rotten childhood.

Before long, Marilyn, a talented singer, was given a screen test by 20th Century Fox executive Ben Lyon, who set her on the path to movie stardom. It was 1950 film *Asphalt Jungle*, in which Monroe rocks an off-the-shoulder black dress that launched her career and position as the world's number one pin-up. Three years later when *Gentlemen Prefer Blondes* was released, she was officially the world's number one sex symbol.

"Give a girl the right shoes and she can conquer the world."

Who do we have to thank for her style? Dress-maker Billy Travilla (of her cream pleated dress billowing over subway fame) helped Marilyn define her ultra-feminine look throughout the 1950s. Her signature became the strapless, backless and cleavage-revealing dresses she sometimes had to lie down to get into.

Marilyn frequently called on the smouldering power of the LBD – the slinky black cocktail dress with long silk gloves and strings of pearls became one of her most enduring looks.

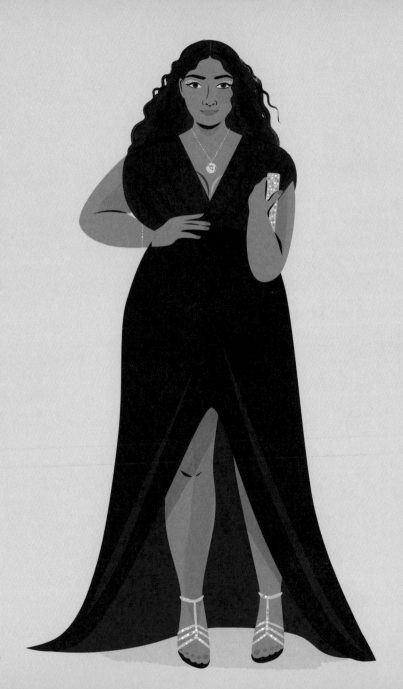

Chiffon V-neck Gown

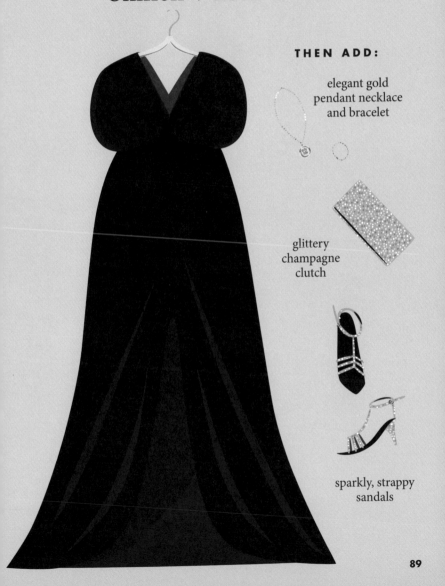

THEN ADD:

elegant gold
pendant necklace
and bracelet

glittery
champagne
clutch

sparkly, strappy
sandals

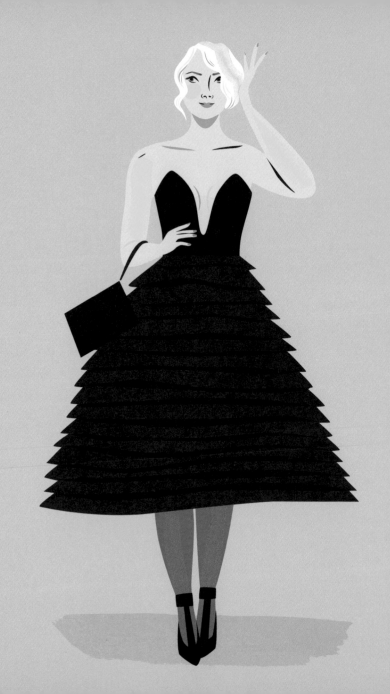

Structured, Tiered Party Dress

THEN ADD:

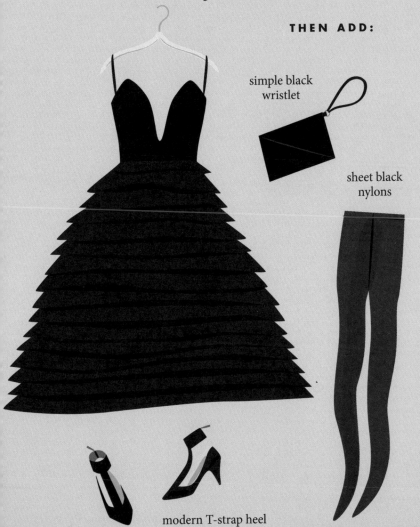

simple black wristlet

sheet black nylons

modern T-strap heel

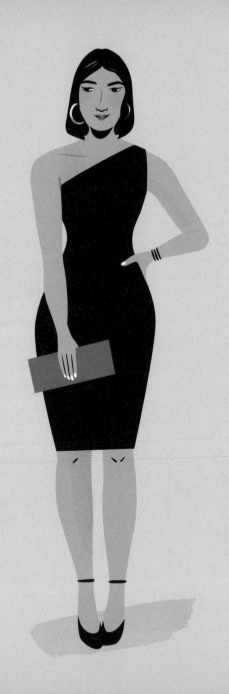

One-shoulder Cocktail Dress

THEN ADD:

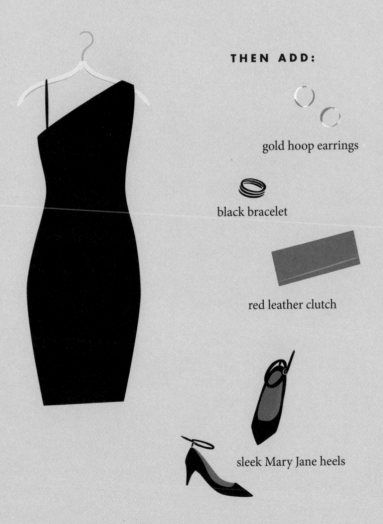

gold hoop earrings

black bracelet

red leather clutch

sleek Mary Jane heels

TOP BRANDS

From designer classics to mid-market originals, each of these brands nails the LBD to perfection. You'll find a multitude of ideas here to suit your style and pocket. Enjoy!

Alexander Wang

San Francisco-born Wang creates understated clothes that ooze the off-duty model vibe. Count on Wang to deliver modern interpretations on the LBD each season including reworkings of the 1990s spaghetti-strap slip and classic shift dress. Walk his way for conceptual shapes and edgy details that will garner compliments.

@alexanderwangny

Chanel

The classic French fashion house, launched by Gabrielle 'Coco' Chanel in 1910, is now under the helm of artistic director Virginie Viard, who worked closely with former creative director, Karl Lagerfeld. Viard has fast made her mark by staying true to the brand values albeit with a modern and extremely wearable twist ensuring Chanel is still the place to go for the ultimate designer LBD.

@chanelofficial

Givenchy

Ever since Hubert de Givenchy (1927–2018) established his fashion house in 1952, the label has been adored for its striking silhouettes and power-packed simplicity. With Audrey Hepburn as his muse, Givenchy created some of the most iconic black dresses of the last century. Now under creative direction of Claire Waight Keller, who designed Meghan Markle's dreamy wedding gown, Givenchy continues to deliver some of the most alluring LBDs around.

@givenchyofficial

Isabel Marant

French designer Isabel Marant, who established her label in 1994, has that *je ne sais quois* ability to know what women want to wear. It's all in the detail – Marant knows exactly how much to drape, embellish and pleat. Say *salut* to her more affordable Etoile diffusion line for wearable-yet-punchy little black shirt dresses and cocktails frocks you'll want to wear and wear.

@isabelmarant

Mother of Pearl

Creative director Amy Powney is putting sustainability at the forefront of this niche east London-based label. Taking inspiration from masculine tailoring, her collection features black dresses made from recycled fabrics in contemporary cuts with fun embellishments, like giant pearls or oversized golden buttons down one side. Chic.

@MotherofPearl

Roland Mouret

Born in a French hillside village just outside Lourdes, Mouret is a self-taught designer who made his name in London in the late 1999s and designed his career-defining, body-accentuating LBD, the Galaxy dress in 2005. His mastery of draping and love of the female form have won him legions of fashion-savvy fans including Carey Mulligan, Claire Danes and Maggie Gyllenhaal.

Sandro

Moroccan-born Evelyne Chetrite moved to Paris as a teen and worked in a vintage shop at the weekends. It was here she got inspired to work as a stylist. She met like-minded Didier and they opened their first store in the Marais in 1984. Since then his label has garnered a loyal following among celebs like Gigi Hadid, Kate Moss and the Duchess of Cambridge, who love the easy urban vibe and simple, modern variations of the LBD like the knitted mini dress or studded wrap.

@sandroparis

Rotate Birger Christensen

This Copenhagen-based brand, designed by stylists Jeanette Madsen and Thora Valdimars,

excels at chic, wearable black dresses. The kind you dream of but can't usually find. The style-savvy pair have become known for creating frocks with billowing sleeves, short hemlines, sheer fabrics and tactile textures, each season delivering a clutch of party-ready LBDs. Sass factor: 11/10.

@rotatebirgerchristensen

Stella McCartney

Brit fashion designer Stella McCartney OBE, (b. 1971), is a life-long vegetarian, making her chic and effortlessly modern takes on the black dress, the obvious choice for meat-free fashionistas. Known for her feminine-yet-empowering cuts, Stella is always sure to create elegant new variations on the black dress whether with full-length red carpet appeal or short and sweet daytime outfits, there's a style to suit you.

@stellamccartney

The Row

Childhood actors-turned-fashion-designers, twins Ashley Olsen and Mary-Kate Olsen, know how to throw an outfit together. Their label, The Row, mimics their own effortless style, with reworkings of the classic LBD from the shift to the 90s slip.

@therow

THE ART OF THE BLACK DRESS

First published in 2020 by Hardie Grant Books,
an imprint of Hardie Grant Publishing

Hardie Grant Books (UK)
52-54 Southwark Street
London SE1 1UN

Hardie Grant Books (Australia)
Ground Floor, Building 1
658 Church Street
Melbourne, VIC 3121

hardiegrantbooks.com

British Library Cataloguing-in-Publication Data. A catalogue
record for this book is available from the British Library.

ISBN: 978-1-78488-278-5
10 9 8 7 6 5 4 3 2 1

Publishing Director Kate Pollard
Editor: Eila Purvis
Illustrator: Libby VanderPloeg
Art Direction: Libby VanderPloeg

Colour Reproduction by p2d
Printed and bound in China by Leo Paper Products Ltd.